I0766274

DISCLAIMER AND TERMS OF USE AGREEMENT:

(Please Read This Before Using This Report)

This information is not presented by a medical practitioner and is for educational and informational purposes only. The content is not intended to be a substitute for professional medical advice, diagnosis, or treatment. Always seek the advice of your physician or other qualified health provider with any questions you may have regarding a medical condition. Never disregard professional medical advice or delay in seeking it because of something you have read.

Since natural and/or dietary supplements are not FDA approved, they must be accompanied by a two-part disclaimer on the product label: that the statement has not been evaluated by FDA and that the product is not intended to "diagnose, treat, cure or prevent any disease.

The author and publisher of this course and the accompanying materials have used their best efforts in preparing this course. The author and publisher make no representation or warranties with respect to the accuracy, applicability, fitness, or completeness of the contents of this course. The information contained in this course is strictly for educational purposes. Therefore, if you wish to apply ideas contained in this course, you are taking full responsibility for your actions.

The author and publisher disclaim any warranties (express or implied), merchantability, or fitness for any particular purpose. The author and publisher shall in no event be held liable to any party for any direct, indirect, punitive, special, incidental or other consequential damages arising directly or indirectly from any use of this material, which is provided "as is", and without warranties.

As always, the advice of a competent legal, tax, accounting, medical or other professional should be sought. The author and publisher do not warrant the performance, effectiveness or applicability of any sites listed or linked to in this course.

All links are for information purposes only and are not warranted for content, accuracy or any other implied or explicit purpose.

This report is © Copyrighted. **No part of this may be copied, or changed in any format, or used in any way other than what is outlined within this course under any circumstances. Violators would be prosecuted severely.**

<u>Contents</u>

Bad Breath In Dogs

What Is Bad Breath?

There are over 90 million people who suffer from simple bad breath or from more severe halitosis. For most people the cause of their bad breath will emanate from their teeth, gums, and tongue. The bad odor will come from bacteria in the mouth that is the result of food particles left in the mouth after eating. Poor dental habits can also be a major contributing cause of bad breath. Decay in the mouth will produce a sulphur compound which leaves behind a bad smell.

If you have bad breath you'll want to take a look at your oral hygiene habits. When you brush your teeth make sure that you also brush your tongue, the inside of your cheeks, and the roof of your mouth. You want to be sure to remove all the food particles and bacteria from your mouth. You'll also want to make sure that you floss your teeth to remove any food particles that are trapped between your teeth. Use a mouthwash as a temporary solution to your bad breath, however if the problem is still there make sure that you talk to your dentist to see if you have gum disease or tooth decay.

Bad breath can also occur for other reasons that include a dry mouth, diabetes, infection, liver problems, or kidney failure. Smoking is another contributing factor. Many cancer patients will find that they have a dry mouth after they have undergone radiation therapy. Lack of saliva in the mouth can lead to bad breath since food particles won't be washed away. Other reasons why you may experience bad breath include stress, dieting, your age, hormonal problems, and snoring.

If you have an odor that emanates from the back of your mouth you may have post-nasal drip. Post-nasal drip occurs when the mucus that is secreted from your nose moves into your throat. The mucus then gets stuck on your tongue and this can produce a foul smell.

The number one thing that you need to keep mouth odors under control is an ample amount of saliva. Saliva is needed to wash away the bacteria and food particles that become stuck in your mouth. As you sleep the amount of saliva that is produced will lessen. This is why most people wake up with some level of morning breath. To get rid of morning breath you simply need to brush and floss your teeth so that the odor is washed away. Eating a morning meal is another way to get rid of morning breath since this will get the saliva flowing once again.

Bad Breath Can Damage Your Career

Not only can bad breath affect your social life, it can also have a negative impact on your career and job prospects. If you want to get the job that you really want you might want to brush your teeth more often and stay away from the coffee. This is because, as some studies show, people who have bad breath are less likely to be considered for a job than people with sweet smelling breath.

If you think that you have bad breath **there are some things that you can focus on** to remedy the matter such as:

- Take more care brushing your teeth. Make sure that you brush your gums, the inside of your cheeks, your tongue, and the roof of your mouth.
- Floss between your teeth at least once each day. You want to make sure that all the food particles are removed from your mouth and from between your teeth.
- Drink plenty of water and other liquids so that your mouth stays wet. Saliva will help to flush out your mouth and can bring you relief from bad breath before it starts.
- Avoid drinking coffee; coffee leaves a distinctive smell in your mouth and can also cause dryness.
- Take the time to clean out your mouth each time that you eat particularly after eating meat, fish, or milk products.
- See your dentist regularly to make sure that you don't have gum problems or tooth decay.
- Use a tongue cleaner to keep your tongue free of bacteria.
- Chew sugarless gum after you eat, particularly if you can't find the time to brush your teeth right away.
- Snack on fresh vegetables like carrots and celery.

Many employers say that bad breath is a very unattractive feature in a potential employee. The only other two unattractive features are body odor and a person who is dressed without care. Employers want to know that the employees they hire are neat and tidy.

Bad breath is a taboo subject that many people avoid taking about. The basic feeling is "if I don't think about it, I don't have it". However, it's important that you recognize whether or not you have bad breath so that you can take the steps necessary to relieve this problem. If you

How To Win Your War Against Bad Breath

have a job interview planned in the near future you're going to want to know whether or not you need to focus on your dental hygiene a little bit more than you usually do. This is especially true if you're applying for a job where you'll be spending a lot of time talking with customers or other employees.

How To Determine If You Have Bad Breath

If you suspect that you have bad breath you'll want to try and determine what type of bad breath you have so that you can take steps to cure it. Bad breath can come under three categories: (1) morning breath, (2) temporary bad breath, and (3) persistent bad breath.

There **are ways of deciding whether you have bad breath** so that you can find a remedy:

- If you find your gums bleed when you brush or floss your teeth it is almost certain that you have bad breath as well.
- Inspect your gums to see if they look red and swollen in places; if they do, it is likely you have bad breath.
- It is sometimes suggested that you can detect your own bad breath by breathing out through your mouth into a paper bag and then breathing in rapidly from the bag through your nose. You might catch a smell of your bad breath by using this method, but usually it does not work because your nose is so used to your own breath smell.
- Put your tongue out as far as you can. Then lick your upper arm or the inner surface of your wrist. Wait four seconds and then smell where you licked.
- Buy a BreathAlert device from the pharmacy. You breathe into the battery-operated device and it gives a reading in terms of one of four grades from no bad breath to strong bad breath.
- Put a piece of gauzy cloth on your tongue, as far back as you can without gagging. Wait for a few moments. Take out the gauze, let it dry and then sniff it.
- If you are a smoker you probably have smoker's breath.
- Ask your dentist or dental hygienist; they are very used to being asked this question.

Bad breath can come about from a variety of sources all the way from the foods that you eat to a medical problem. Your dentist will be able to tell you if your bad breath is the result of tooth decay or gum problems. If your bad breath is caused by a dental condition it should disappear once you have been treated by your dentist.

If you find that you get bad breath after eating certain foods you may want to avoid these foods when you know that you're going to be out in public or spending time with your loved one. Common foods to avoid include garlic, curry spices, cabbages, and alcohol.

Do You Have Chronic Bad Breath?

Many people around us have the problem of chronic bad breath. This is a condition where you have bad breath constantly which will interrupt you badly from talking, no matter where, either in your work place or your personal life. Chronic bad breath may be caused because of the presence of some oral bacterial infection or a medical condition of some sort. Chronic bad breath can create a negative impact among the people you deal with day to day. As a matter of fact, it is very important for you to find out whether you have chronic bad breath or not. If you think you are putting off people with your chronic bad breath, then consider the following things which will help you decide if your bad breath will become a problem or not.

The most basic thing that can be done by you to find out whether you have chronic bad breath or not, is by checking if you have a bad taste in your mouth. This is mainly due to the decay of food particles that is left back in your mouth after having any food. As long as you clean your tongue and teeth properly after having food you will not have bad breath and if you have and it is left unchecked then this results in chronic bad breath. This can be avoided by brushing up your teeth regularly after having your food whether it is breakfast\lunch\dinner\supper. Another basic thing is if you have a white or yellow coating in your tongue it may lead to chronic bad breath. This can also be avoided by brushing or scrapping off regularly. If you allow it to build up continuously there is a chance of creating bad breath.

Other ways through which you can find out if you have chronic bad breath or not are:
When you stand among your dear or near ones and if they step back away from you as soon as you start talking or if they offer you any breath freshening gum or a breath mint before they start talking with you is a clue that you can pick up on, this would indicate that you have chronic bad breath. If this event occurs regularly then you have a serious issue as many people will not actually come out and say it. Most people around us are much too polite to mention this directly and will only indicate subtly by offering us a mint or a gum.

To conclude in order to avoid chronic bad breath brush or scrape your tongue and teeth regularly after having food and visit a dentist doctor once in a while. Avoiding chronic bad breath can lead you to more joyful interactions with your dear or near ones or even with other people. People would stop offering you a gum\mint and will not avoid you from their conversations.

Bad Breath – What Are The Causes of Bad Breath?

You must definitely have come across at least one person who suffered with chronic bad breath. The reasons for this could be a poor diet, or a bad diet which causes bad breath or a health condition that is the cause of this problem. Various people have different causes for bad breath and it differs from one to the other. Investigations by a medical practitioner will give an insight into the exact health problem and the root cause of bad breath. Apart from dental conditions it could also be because of a gum disease, a throat infection or tonsillitis too.

Food habits the cause of bad breath

What you eat is a very probable cause of the bad breath as the mouth is the beginning of the alimentary canal. Sometimes the odor of the food remains in the mouth for a long time and no amount of brushing the teeth or gargling can get rid of this. Some foods give an extra bad odor like onions and garlic, and alcohol and tobacco also contribute to this bad odor. However, there are some things that will help to clear the breath like mint, lettuce, parsley and other greens. No matter what you eat ensure that it is washed thoroughly and that it is not the cause for indigestion. Indigestion is another cause of bad breath.

Oral Hygiene is important

Uppermost on the list of avoiding bad breath is the oral hygiene that you maintain. You must brush your teeth after each meal and floss your teeth at least once a day. After every meal or even a snack make sure that you clear all the particles from your mouth and the crevices of your teeth. Any food particles that remain here will be a cause for the increase of bacteria which gives rise to bad breath. So make sure that you keep your mouth absolutely clean all the time. Once this is neglected it will affect your dental conditions which will decay and deteriorate giving further cause for bad breath.

See a medical practitioner

Once you have gone over all the possible causes of bad breath and have eliminated all, then the last resort is to see a doctor to get the final diagnosis for bad breath. Whatever the cause, it is best to ensure ones own personal hygiene and maintain a clean and healthy way of living. This itself will be sufficient enough to help you to avoid bad breath in future.

Halitosis And Bad Personal Habits

It is relatively simple to avoid bad breath. Although it is commonly known that mouth fresheners are instantaneously active at keeping away bad breath, long lasting benefits can be obtained by simple acts of good hygiene. In the majority of cases, halitosis is caused as a result of nothing more than laziness or carelessness. It may not always be possible to brush after every meal when dining outside your home and this inevitably leads to bad breath especially if your meal is spicy. Likewise, although inconvenient, flossing removes particles of food stuck between the teeth.

Not every cause of halitosis is beyond one's control. Over time, people could develop bad hygiene like not brushing or flossing before going to bed or they may not drink as much water as is needed. Not visiting the dentist regularly will also lead to the spurting and thriving of bacterial colonies inside the gums and can become extremely difficult to eliminate completely. There may be some bacteria that are beneficial to health, but the bad ones need to be kept at bay. By and large, good personal hygiene with regular dental check-ups should be enough to prevent the main causes of halitosis from taking root.

Metabolic Cause for Halitosis

Diabetes could be symptom free during its early phases. Surveys have shown that a large number of people in many different countries suffer from diabetes, without ever being aware of it. This causes a build up of ketones in the blood. Ketones are exceptionally malodorous chemicals produced when the body uses fat instead of carbohydrates as a source of energy. Ketones are generally excreted from the body in sweat, urine and the exhaled air. Halitosis caused by ketones cannot be cured by simply a dentist alone. As a result, dentists may refer a patient to a general physician, when no oral causes of halitosis can be found. It is also probable, as a high blood pressure leads to deficiency of the immune system, that diabetes and bacterial infections are related as well.

A sudden change of the type of food taken could also result in bad breath. Fasting and a high protein, low carbohydrate diet also leads to ketosis. In the bodies of people hoping to lose weight or boost musculature, more fat is burned as a source of energy and this leads to a build up of high levels of ketones in the blood which eventually finds its way to the lungs. This is the reason for special diets being prepared by experts for specific individuals.

Bad Breath Cause - Common Causes For Bad Breath

The most common bad breath

For the majority of the people bad breath is a problem when they wake up in the morning, but this is ok once they have brushed their teeth and cleaned their mouths thoroughly. However, as the day goes on, the bad breath may be there again and people may be staying away from you and avoiding close contact with you.

Bad breath after a meal

If your meal has been heavily garnished with garlic you will find that your breath smells of garlic too, similarly if you have eaten onions or smoked cigarettes. Alcohol also leaves its mark on your breath and makes it positively unpleasant for anyone to approach too close to you.

Another cause for halitosis

Camouflaging the bad breath with breath fresheners will or mouth sprays is a temporary effect that will mask the bad breath only for a short time. If the main cause of the halitosis or bad breath is not cured or dealt with then nothing can clear it permanently. So you have to get down to the root of the problem literally and cure that first. It may be poor dental hygiene or teeth that have to be seen to, so this you will have to visit your dentist. Even if your digestion is affected by the food that you have eaten, your can have bad breath.

Chronic bad breath

There may be some people who maintain an excellent oral hygiene but still suffer from the worst possible halitosis. Chronic bad breath is when a person has foul odor from the nose and the mouth at all times. Unfortunately as these people have very clean oral hygiene they do not know what to do about this embarrassing condition.

Cause of bad breath

Bacterium is the most common underlying problem that causes bad breath. This is because of the food particles that get left behind in the mouth after a meal and which the bacterium starts feeding on. To fight this problem a thorough cleansing of the mouth after every meal and with a proper tooth brush would help. The back of the teeth should not be neglected and the toothbrush should have bristles that reach in between the teeth too. So no area is left neglected and all food particles are removed.

How To Win Your War Against Bad Breath

The proper way to brush your teeth

To make sure that you have brushed your mouth very thoroughly you should take at least 5 minutes to do so and make sure that your brush has reached all the crevices and corners. If you leave any areas unattended this would be a cause for bad breath.

Another fact that you should keep in mind is that all toothpastes are not alike. Some would only worsen the problem instead of helping it. Toothpastes that have peroxide or baking soda in them are the best to use. These two ingredients will make a lot of difference to bad breath and give you more self confidence when you are inter acting with people.

Authoritative Answers For The Common Question: What Causes Bad Breath?

Halitosis or bad breath is a condition where the person has bad breath. This could be for several reasons and for those who have it, it is an eternal question as to what causes bad breath so that they can avoid it and at least control it.

Eating certain foods affects the breath

Some foods have strong odors like garlic and onions and this lingers on in the mouth after a meal. Using mouth fresheners and a thorough brushing of the teeth may not do much to get rid of this kind of an odor and in any case the relief would be temporary as this odor is exhaled through the breath even after the food is digested. However, even food is not the only reason that causes halitosis, though food particles that are caught between the teeth usually cause bad breath because of the bacteria that thrives on these particles. Some times a medical condition could be responsible for this problem.

Some simple solutions for bad breath

There is no hard and fast condition that causes bad breath and if it is persistent it is always better to consult a medical practitioner to find out the reason. It is good to have a regular dental check up and see to the condition of one's teeth and general oral conditions. Sometimes it may be necessary to do some blood tests to see what the underlying cause of bad breath could be. There could be some serious problem in the system also and it is better to have this diagnosed instead of taking things into ones own hands. What ever the problem one can take care of this to some extent by keeping the mouth clean at all times. Wrong eating habits and an unhealthy diet can also cause bad breath without any health conditions involved. So ensure that you eat a balanced diet and there should be little cause to worry about bad breath.

Good habits

If there is no serious health problem then it would do to have hygienic habits and avoid bad breath. Staying away from tobacco is another thing that would help your breath. The basic simple facts are to brush your teeth after each meal and to floss them regularly whether we are adults or children and avoid getting chronic bad breath.

Bad Breath And Acidic Foods

Studies show that acidic foods can cause some people to have bad breath. If you've tried other methods of getting rid of bad breath, and find that you've not been successful, you might want to eliminate highly acidic foods from your diet to see what the result is in regards to foul odors. Fighting bad breath often means trying two or more solutions until you find the right one for you.

Acids will help the bacteria in your mouth to reproduce at a faster rate. You need to neutralize the acids in your mouth so that sulphur compounds are discouraged from growing. The easiest way that you can do this is by eliminating certain foods from your diet.

Coffee is probably one of the first food items that you should stop using. Both regular coffee and decaf coffee has high acid levels. Substitute your morning coffee with a cup of tea since tea is much less acidic. Another beverage that you should avoid drinking is tomato juice.

There are other juices that also contain high levels of acid which you'll want to eliminate for a time so that you can see if your bad breath disappears or is eased. These juices include orange juice, pineapple juice, and grapefruit juice. High acid fruits should also be avoided so that you can neutralize your mouth.

Bad Breath And High Protein Foods

Foods that are high in protein can make your bad breath much worse. This is because some high protein foods cause sulphur compounds to grow at a very fast rate. And for you this means an environment in your mouth that is ideal for bacteria to grow and multiply.

There are some foods that contribute more to the production of sulphur compounds than other foods. These foods come under the category of "high protein/amino acid foods. Milk, cheese, and other diary products are at the top of the list when it comes to high protein foods that you should avoid. If you are lactose intolerant you'll definitely want to stop eating dairy products since these foods will be around longer for bacteria to thrive on.

Fish is very high in protein and should be avoided completely for a time being to see if your bad breath improves. Substitute other protein foods, such as tofu, so that you're sure to get the amount of protein that you need each day.

When it comes to acidic foods you'll want to avoid coffee until you can determine if your bad breath is caused by the foods that you ingest. Coffee, whether it's regular or decaf, contains large amounts of acids. It's these acids that help bacteria to reproduce at a fast rate. Coffee can also leave your mouth with a bitter taste that can contribute to bad breath.

Dry Mouth And Bad Breath

If you have a dry mouth, you'll have less saliva. And less saliva in your mouth can lead to bad breath. **Saliva is very important** to dental and oral hygiene **since it performs the following functions:**

- Saliva provides necessary enzymes which are needed to digest your food.
- Saliva helps to stabilize the pH levels in your mouth, which in effect control the amount of acids that are present.
- Saliva provides adequate levels of oxygen which are needed to keep the tissues in your mouth fresh and healthy.

Dry mouth, otherwise known as Xerostomia, means that you have less saliva. This means that there will be less oxygen in your mouth. When oxygen is lacking an anaerobic environment will be created which is perfect for the production of bacteria. Bacteria in the mouth will create sulphur gases which will give you bad breath and also leave a bad taste in your mouth.

The shape of your tongue can also determine whether or not you have bad breath. The rougher that your tongue is the more likely you'll have bad breath since there will be more grooves in which bacteria can hide. Everyone has a specific shape and texture of tongue which can be an inherited factor in the freshness of your breath.

Some people will have a hairy tongue. This means that the papillae, the fibers of the tongue, are longer than average. These long fibers can trap in those bacteria that produce foul smelling sulphurs.

If you scrape your tongue or brush it extra hard to combat bad breath you may develop what is known as "burning tongue syndrome". This syndrome occurs when you develop sensitivity to certain conditions such as hot, cold, or acidic foods. If you have a tongue that is sensitive you'll want to stay away from mouthwashes and oral rinses that have an alcohol base.

Once you know that bad breath and a dry mouth go hand in hand you can take steps to make sure that your mouth remains wet with an ample amount of saliva. Chewing on gum throughout the day can help to keep the saliva flowing but make sure that you use sugarless gum so that

you avoid tooth decay. You can also try keeping a bottle of water with you at all times so that you can wet your whistle once you feel that your mouth is getting too dry. Bad breath can be an unpleasant part of your life until you learn some of the tricks of avoiding it.

Methamphetamine Can Cause Bad Breath

How do you find out whether your kid is using it?

One of the earliest, and common signs that your kid maybe using Methamphetamine, is bad breath. The breath smells like a foul smelling chemical. Brushing the teeth vigorously and any number of times will not help in taking away the bad breath. Apart from this look at the eyes for signs too, the pupils will be dilated. Another sign is very dry cracked lips, nose bleeds because of dry nostrils and symptoms of sinus as this drug can be smoked or snorted.

Outward symptoms of Methamphetamine use

The person using this drug looses appetite to the point of becoming anorexic. Insomnia or not being able to sleep, overly anxious, aggressive, a nervous nature and chattering incessantly along with an overall hyperactive attitude are all signs of the use of this drug.

The person may try desperately to get rid of the bad breath by using a lot of mouth washes, breath fresheners, lozenges and breath sprays but to no avail, nothing can get rid of this bad breath that is brought on by the use of methamphetamine. No matter what is done to camouflage the use of this drug, these signs cannot be eliminated. You should keep a watch for any signs and changed behavior of your child and put a stop to this harmful habit before it is too late to help the child.

Life threatening side effects of the drug

Apart from bad breath there are other life threatening effects on health. So it is up to you as a parent to watch out for any of these signs and help your child. Other life threatening symptoms are raised blood pressure and heart rate that could prove to be fatal if care is not taken in the beginning itself to stop the use of this drug. The blood vessels to the brain get damaged and the person could have a stroke and die.

Even after the drug is stopped there will be changes in the behavior and psychotic symptoms in the person. The parent should watch out for bad breath and ask the child what the problem is. They should not back off or be afraid of asking the child about all this as it is only going to help your child in the long run. Parent should monitor the changes in their child so that they are aware of what is happening in the child's life at all times.

What To Do About Bad Breath

Dealing with a person who has bad breath can often prove to be a problem. The person who is in an intimate conversation with a second person may find it horrible to suddenly realize that the other person has bad breath. This in turn may also evoke the listener to make facial expressions that communicate disgust. He or she may feel nauseous and may even avoid talking to that person again. This sort of response is instinctive and completely involuntary. The easiest way to deal with bad breath is to get away from it as fast as possible.

To deal with something like bad breath is a difficult issue. However, it is also important that the issue is dealt with all together, even if it is a personal issue or regarding someone else like a friend, relative or colleague.

HOW ONE CAN DEAL WITH IT ONESELF:

The easiest way to deal with bad breath is to take care of one's personal hygiene, especially that pertaining to the teeth and oral hygiene at large. This helps to a certain extent. Often being lazy or not caring much about these aspects costs one his or her self esteem and respect. It can lead to the gradual decline of one's self respect as well. People who are aware of their bad breath can seek medical help like that of a dentist's, if they are unable to handle it by themselves. The best way to get rid of laziness and ignorance is to be aware of the fact that your ignorance can make others suffer as well.

HOW TO INFORM OTHERS:

What do you do when you come across a person with bad breath? You wouldn't even think about informing the person. What we often fail to realize is that addressing the issue is the most important step to be taken. Starting off with this sort of a personal conversation can be difficult. It so happens that bad breath can be the result of some medical problem and by informing the concerned person of the issue, we can save that person's life from danger in extreme circumstances.

Wondering what you can do? The easiest way to bring the talk up is to offer that person a piece of gum or mint and then start the conversation. Another option is to give a general talk about bad breath and then offer the person the gum or mint. Most of the people can comprehend the

How To Win Your War Against Bad Breath

hint. However, some people may even need direct statements regarding their bad breath. All of these can be hard and difficult to implement, but are things that have to be done all the same.

<u>Curing Bad Breath</u>

Before you can fix bad breath you have to have some idea of what is causing it. In about 80 to 90 percent of the cases of bad breath the culprit will be something that is in your mouth. Usually this will be nothing more serious that a mouth that is dirty. Plaque is one of the leading causes of bad breath. Plaque is an invisible layer of bacteria that is present in your mouth. Bacteria can often cause bad breath. Other dental factors, such as gum disease and cavities, can also cause bad breath. Bad breath can also be caused by something that is in the gastrointestinal tract or in the lungs. Systemic infections can also be a factor.

Strong foods are often a leading contributor to bad breath. For instance, a meal that has garlic in it can cause breath that is strong and foul. Other strong foods include onions and curry spices. These foods are carried along in the bloodstream and are then exhaled through the lungs. Alcohol and tobacco are other causes of bad breath. There are some health problems that can cause bad breath in some people, such as diabetes or sinus infections.

There are some things that you can do to keep your breath as fresh as possible:

- Keep your mouth clean. Try to brush at least twice each day and floss at least once. Bacteria and food that is left in your mouth and between your teeth will cause bad breath.
- Brush your tongue. Bacteria left on your tongue can also contribute to bad breath.
- Avoid a dry mouth. Saliva will help to keep your mouth clean since it acts as a natural antibacterial and helps to wash away food particles from your mouth.
- Rinse your mouth after eating. Rinsing with water can help to remove some of the food particles that are left in your mouth after you eat. A quick rinse can help to fight bad breath.
- Chew on parsley. Although chewing on parsley won't cure you of bad breath but it will mask the smell for a short period of time. Spearmint will work just as well.
- Fight plague. Eating foods that help to fight plague can also help you fight bad breath. Good food choices include peanuts, carrots, cheese, and celery.

The above tips will help to keep your breath sweet smelling. If you're looking for a long term solution you need to find out the cause is behind your bad breath.

Finding the Right Bad Breath Remedy

There are few things in life more embarrassing than bad breath. Everybody afflicted with this condition is searching for that one elusive cure which can cure them of their condition and make life a lot easier to live. Unfortunately, remedies are not exactly straightforward.

If you are one of those many souls searching for a cure, the place you are most likely to find that cure is most definitely a medical professional. Your physician can give you a lot more personalized information on which remedy would suit you the best and help you choosing in one as he knows your body much better than anyone else. In case you need a cure immediately, here are a couple of them. These may or may not work for you but it is important that you actively search for the cure that would suit you best to ensure that all future encounters with other people is not an embarrassing one and you are in your comfort zone.

Drink Water!

The reason for bad breath, excluding improper brushing and flossing, is probably a dry mouth. In case you don't drink enough fluids, it's a good bet that the reason for your foul smelling breath is the want for moisture inside your mouth. Drinking enough water is vital for good health, with a bad breath only one reason to make sure you drink enough.

In case you find it difficult to drink water as such, try to eat a lot of fruits. Fruits are full of water and are a guaranteed way of getting more fluids into your body. This is an ideal way to start changing your diet which is the second of the remedies already mentioned.

Change your Diet

Eating a lot of meat instead of vegetables and fruits can also lead to a malodorous breath. Staying off high protein meat and eating more fresh food is an ideal remedy for those who already brush and floss regularly and drink enough water to keep their mouths moist and get the required amount of fluids for their body, but still suffer from bad breath.

How To Win Your War Against Bad Breath

Next time, skip the juicy steak and opt for a healthy salad instead. It is one of those rare bad breath remedies that actually work. You won't know if it is effective till you have tried it out for yourself. A bad breath is not as difficult as most of us think it is to cure.

Bad Breath Solutions

When it comes to bad breath the natural remedies that most people think of are to improve on their brushing and flossing routine. However, a well balanced diet can also play a big role in eliminating your bad breath problems. A digestive system that works efficiently can greatly reduce the amount of bacteria in your body that are the cause of odors.

Acidophilus is something that you should make sure you have enough of in your diet. Studies show that an imbalance of bacteria in your intestines can contribute to your bad breath. Increasing the amount of acidophilus in your body can be achieved by eating more yogurt which is rich in live cultures.

Vitamin C can aid in protecting your gums from damage to the cells as well as help in speeding up healing. Bad breath can often be caused by gums that are in poor health. Good sources of Vitamin C include cabbage, red peppers, strawberries, oranges, and kiwi fruit.

Try to replace some of the animal protein that you eat with high fiber foods such as vegetables and fruits. Vegetables and fruits can help to cleanse your breath because they are high in fiber and have large amounts of enzymes. During your day munch on raw vegetables and fruit such as apples, pears, carrots, and parsley sprigs. Parsley is a natural breath freshener because it contains chlorophyll. Chlorophyll is a chemical that keeps plants green and is considered to be a natural breath freshener.

Drink at **least eight glasses of water** each day so that your mouth is always moist. You'll also be flushing out the germs and bacteria that can gather in your mouth from particles of food. Visit your dentist to be sure that gum disease or tooth decay isn't an underlying factor of your bad breath. Keep in mind that Vitamin C is good for preventing gum disease.

One last thing that you can do is eat fiber rich foods to fight constipation. Studies show that regular bowel movements will remove those toxins from your body that can cause bad breath. When you eat large amounts of meat you absorb a lot of bacteria into your bloodstream which then passes into your lungs and is then exhaled as bad breath. High sources of fiber include brown rice, peas, figs, dried bean, wheat products, and prunes.

How To Win Your War Against Bad Breath

Eating a **balanced diet** is a good way to make sure that your body is in good condition and working as it should. This alone can help you to eliminate your bad breath.

How To Cure Bad Breath

Causes of bad breath

Bad breath is usually caused by bacteria that is formed in your mouth and feeds upon the food particles that are left between the teeth after a meal. The best way to ensure that your mouth is clean after a meal is to brush your teeth and try and do this after every meal to prevent the bacteria from building up. This way you can prevent getting bad breath.

Food that is stuck in the teeth allows the bacteria to grow and makes this a chronic problem if not tackled immediately. This problem is more with meat eaters than with those who are vegetarian only. The bacteria thrive on the meat that is left in the mouth, between the teeth after a meal.

The best ways to keep your mouth clean and avoid bad breath

The plaque formation on the teeth is another area where the bacteria thrive and are the cause for bad breath. The plaque can also get under the gums and if not treated or seen to immediately could cause grave dental problems. Brushing your teeth thoroughly several times a day will get rid of any problem that creates bad breath and can eliminate it altogether. It is very important to floss your teeth everyday. This way the plaque is not given a chance to settle on your teeth and below the gums.

Another important method to get rid of bad breath is to prevent the bacteria from getting any food and multiplying in your mouth. The best way is to ensure that there are no food particles left in your mouth after a meal. Obviously brushing your teeth and flossing them after every meal is the key factor to a clean mouth.

See the dentist

If you find that none of this is helping you to get rid of the bad breath then it is definitely time for you to see a dentist. The dentist could do a thorough cleaning of the mouth and also see if there is any other underlying cause for the bad breath. Ask for advice on how to maintain your mouth the same way as it was after a professional cleaning and learn how to maintain it like that always.

The Main Cure For Bad Breath

Have you wondered why people often stay away from you when you talk to them? The reason can be your failure to find an apt cure for bad breath. You may be one among the other million people who suffer from foul breath or halitosis and still unable to find a cure for bad breath. If foul mouth odor is haunting your thoughts, then it is high time you quickly find a cure for bad breath.

BACTERIA -THE REASON FOR HALITOSIS:

Nearly ninety percent of halitosis cases can be attributed to bacteria that dwell in the mouth and a majority of these bacteria commonly gather behind the tongue. Hence to get rid of bad breath, one would have to dislodge these bacteria from their haunts in the mouth and surrounding areas.

Bacteria can multiply at an alarming rate anywhere in your mouth, be it in the crevices between you teeth or on your tongue. This growth is triggered by the passage of food through the mouth. Food particles often tend to remain in the mouth after a meal especially between the teeth or your gum line and the bacteria bloom from them. Bacteria triggered bad breath often begins from here.

DISLODGING THE BACTERIA - HOW?

Regularly brushing is the only way to get rid of unwanted bacterial organisms from your mouth and gum lines. The cure for bad breath often includes brushing properly at least two to three times a day and scraping your tongue as well. The texture of the tongue is the favorite dwelling place of the halitosis causing bacteria. One thing that we often do as a cure for bad breath is the usage of mouth wash or gum which only results in the masking of the odor and in the absence of the mint or the gum, the bad breath persists. On the other hand, brushing and flossing results in the permanent dislodging of the bad breath causing bacteria.

Ignoring your bad breath by just using mint or gum can be a wrong step. Regular brushing and flossing can be the only cure for bad breath. However, if it still seems hard to handle, one can seek professional help like that of a dentist's.

How To Win Your War Against Bad Breath

An effective cure for your bad breath can be a truly liberating experience. Getting rid of halitosis by the regular and appropriate maintenance of oral hygiene can enable you to talk with exuberant confidence. It is said that one among four suffer from bad breath. So hurry and get rid of it if you don't want to be that person.

Bad Breath Remedies For Home Use

Bad breath becomes a social problem for any one who suffers with it. They cannot get close to people without feeling embarrassed and are always aware of this short coming. Some people cannot afford to go to doctors and some just do not like to do so especially, to dentists. For this category of people there are home remedies which could be of some help, maybe not in curing the problem but at least minimizing it to some extent.

Thorough cleaning habits

Keeping good oral hygiene and maintaining clean dental habits is the first remedy. So it is essential to brush your teeth after every meal and floss them at least once a day. If you cannot do this minimal thing then it shows that you are either not aware of the problem or do not want to be bothered with trying to maintain a better oral hygiene. This would be the first step in helping you to get rid of your bad breath.

Eating avocado helps bad breath

This is not a much known fact but eating avocado can reduce bad breath considerably. Of course you should not do the overeating bit too. This fruit is available easily in every grocery store and is effective in controlling the problem of bad breath to quite an extent.

Reduce your intake of protein

If you are conscious of the fact that you have bad breath then you should find out the reason for it too. Maybe you are eating protein rich food like too much of steak or chicken and meat. This definitely increases bad breath. Instead switch over to more vegetables and fresh fruits and see the improvement in your condition. By changing your eating habits you will reduce or even get rid of the bad breath completely.

Start drinking more water

Another common cause of bad breath is a dry mouth. Drinking more water will not only help this but also help many other medical problems too. You can consume water directly or eat a lot of water bearing fruits and juices to increase the quantity of fluid intake on a regular basis. It is advisable to take drinking water in a measured bottle and make it a point to finish this water. In this way you will be aware of the amount of water you have consumed and can try and increase it a little everyday.

Herbal Remedies For Bad Breath

There are many people who swear that herbal remedies work for bad breath. If you suffer from bad breath you might want to try some of the following herbal products to see if you can promote a sweeter breath:

- **Anise**: Anise seeds are a licorice flavored seed that can kill the bacteria in your mouth as well as mask the odor. Other seeds to try include fennel, dill, or cardamom.
- **Cloves**: Cloves are known as a powerful antiseptic. Make yourself a clove mouthwash which you can use twice a day. Place 3 whole cloves into two cups of boiling water. Let this mixture steep for about 20 minutes. Pour the mixture through a strainer and put the liquid into a jar.
- **Lemon**: Take a lemon wedge and sprinkle a little bit of salt on the stop. Suck on the lemon wedge until the juices are gone. This will help to stop bad breath after you've eaten onions or garlic.
- **Parsley**: Try chewing on a few sprigs of parsley. Parsley has been used for thousands of years in the promotion of good smelling breath. Mint works just as well as parsley.
- **Fennel**: There are two ways that you can use fennel to fight bad breath: (1) chew the leaves slowly so that saliva builds up in your mouth, or (2) take a fennel capsule (found in health food stores) and open it up, mixing the contents with baking soda so that you make a paste. Use this paste to brush your teeth, gums, and tongue.

Folk Remedies for Bad Breath

Over the years there have been many folk remedies that are used to combat bad breath. Whether they work or not will be up to you. One of the most popular folk remedies is the use of apple cider vinegar. After each meal swallow a tablespoon of apple cider vinegar either straight or diluted in a glass of water. Not only will this fight your bad breath, it will also aid you in digesting your meal.

Brush your teeth with baking soda to reduce or eliminate bad breath. Baking soda will help to neutralize the acids in your mouth which can promote the growth of bacteria. You can also look for tooth pastes that are made with hydrogen peroxide to achieve the same results. Hydrogen peroxide is also helpful in keeping your sinuses healthy. Infected sinuses can cause you to have bad breath that is very unpleasant. Dilute the hydrogen peroxide (sold in pharmacies at a strength of 3%) with about 50% water. Place about five to ten drops of the solution into each nostril, making sure to inhale deeply.

Gargling with salt water is another way that you can flush out the bacteria in your mouth. You'll also be gargling out food particles and mucus which can lead to bad breath. Make sure that you gargle deep back into your throat so that your tonsils are flushed.

A Simple Cure For Bad Breath With Zantac

Treating the basic cause of the bad breath will help eradicate the problem and the key is to find out the main disorder that is causing this. Digestive problems like acidity can cause bad breath and a simple ant acid will help in getting rid of the bad breath.

Bad breath is caused by peptic ulcers

Some times a certain bacteria in the body can cause other problems like digestive disorders too. A common problem is that of peptic ulcers where the person has reflux and also vomiting. This is also because of the acidity in the stomach and the food remaining undigested giving rise to gasses in the stomach which come up to the mouth. This causes bad breath. However, the cure for this is fairly simple as a drug like Zantac can bring the problem under control and get rid of the bad breath too.

How does Zantac cure bad breath?

Zantac helps in curing the acidity in the stomach which is aggravating the ulcer. With this the heart burn and reflux is reduced and also puts a stop to the odors that emit from these gasses in the stomach. Apart from Zantac an antibiotic may also be prescribed to treat the bacteria in the stomach and the ulcer will also disappear. With this combination in treating the problem the bad breath will be cured also. The main thing is to find out the cause of bad breath and treat it instead of only external solutions.

Consult a doctor for the problem

If a person has any chronic problem with their health it is always advisable to see their personal physician so that they can find out the underlying cause of the problem. Similarly if a person has bad breath accompanied with heart burn and other digestive problems like vomiting then it is better not to try just home remedies but to get expert advice. The doctor will probably have some tests done to diagnose the problem that is causing the bad breath and the heart burn. In case it is confirmed to be a digestive problem then Zantac will help it immediately.

Though Zantac can be procured over the counter it has various strengths and it is better to consult the doctor before buying it for yourself. However, if there is going to be a delay in seeing the doctor then you can start on the medication while waiting for the final

How to Cure British Columbia Bad Breath

Whether you reside in British Columbia or in Timbuktu, bad breath happens to be a real problem. Bad breath affects so many aspects of life such as a person's ability to land a good job, his ability to socialize and make friends, to find that special someone and enjoy a flourishing love life and many other things of a similar character. British Columbia bad breath is only another type of malodorous breath and the only important thing is how you deal with it.

Visit a Specialist

The British Columbia bad breath happens to be notoriously difficult to cure. Most often it becomes necessary to visit a doctor who specializes in British Columbia bad breath who has had a lot of experiencing in treating it to be successfully cured. If you can, you can take the advice of a regular physician or even an intern but in case you don't have those options, visit the dentist and find out if they are able to help you in dealing with this affliction.

Visiting a specialist in British Columbia bad breath is a great way to ensure that you happen to be in the finest shape you could probably be and that happens to pretty important. Healthy teeth and gums form a much bigger part of overall wellbeing than you ever imagined was possible.

Alleviate it on Your Own

In case you are a resident of British Columbia, remember that bad breath there is cured in much the same way as elsewhere. Ensure that your mouth is as hygienic as you could possibly make it by regularly flossing and brushing your teeth the spaces between teeth daily and rinsing your mouth using anti-microbial mouthwash. Apart from successfully curing British Columbia bad breath, these practices also ensure the good health of your gums and teeth which is a vital aspect of ensuring that your body happens to be in the best possible shape.

Do Not Despair

Immaterial of whether you reside in British Columbia or Timbuktu, remember that bad breath is as curable as it is elsewhere. To find the ideal cure for you, you need to realize what part of your

How To Win Your War Against Bad Breath

food or lifestyle causes the malodorous breath and after you have identified the crux of the issue; your chances of completely being cured of bad breath are really good.

Leave Bad Breath Treatment To Your Dentist

Oral fresheners make a lot of good sense. There may be an especially pungent item in the food you eat outside of your home or it could be that you have a soft spot for garlic or onions. It is difficult for family members and friends to work up the courage to inform you that you could be suffering from halitosis but a dentist would have no qualms in doing so. Oral fresheners bought off the shelf without a prescription is not a remedy anyway. Short-term relief is just not enough if the affliction recurs frequently or appears to be unrelated to eating habits.

Any dentist would need to thoroughly examine the internal surfaces of your mouth, in order to find out if you have halitosis, ahead of deciding on a set of treatments to deal with your specific problem. At times, drinking more water or just chewing gum could be enough to do away with the dry mouth problem which concentrates the foul smelling substances while breathing out. Although it is mostly children culpable of unacceptable brushing habits, at times, adults may be careless as well. Regular scraping of the tongue and removing particles of food stuck in between the teeth are some habits which can greatly reduce the occurrence of bad breath. A dentist is capable of removing plaque built up over time, cure gum diseases, and recommend antibiotics to treat bad breath.

Treating bad Breath beyond Your Mouth

Dentists can't treat all halitosis cases by themselves. Disease of the gums may be very entrenched and could require the attention of a specialist. But not all instances of bad breath have their genesis in the mouth. A dentist could send a patient suffering from halitosis to a doctor to help in curing a general cause. Ketones are odorous compounds, which are usually excreted in perspiration, urine and in the exhaled breath too. If a person suffers from diabetes, has not been eating, or if his carbohydrate intake is inadequate, the level of ketones in the blood builds up. As ketosis can be fatal, halitosis could be an indicator of a much more serious medical condition. This is why all cases of chronic bad breath require medical attention.

Thankfully, treatment of bad breath is relatively simple once the basic origin has been identified. But it may re-occur if the patient refuses to follow the recommendations or change his personal habits which caused the problem in the first place. As bad breath can strike at anytime, being cured of it once doesn't mean that it will never recur again. It is ideal to have a family member or a close friend to check regularly and never miss an appointment with your dentist.

Bad Breath - 5 Remedies

While trying to find an effective remedy for malodorous breath, you will need to scrutinize the reason for the bad breath so that it can be treated properly. Malodorous breath is a widely prevalent condition and it's comforting to know that a cure is available and that bad breath could be dealt with effectively.

Some of the major causes of foul smelling breath are foods, oral bacteria, dentures, dry mouth and smoking. Every one of these factors cause either short - term or chronic bad breath. Fortunately, a cure also exists for every one of these conditions.

1. Bacteria in the Mouth

The main cause or bad breath is oral bacteria and they can be completely eradicated by routine and effective flossing and brushing of teeth and routine tongue scraping. Oral bacteria as their name suggests reside in the mouth and the tongue is one of their favorite haunts. You have to remove food residue and plaque from the mouth to ensure that bacteria don't take hold in your mouth. By the adoption of a regular flossing and brushing routine, oral bacteria and the ensuing bad breath could be eliminated completely.

2. Bad Breath Caused by Foods

Food items such as garlic and onions cause bad breath in the short term and this odor can be masked by eating foods like cloves, parsley, and peppermint or fennel seeds. This odor can only be masked as it has its origins in the intestines and you need to wait a whole day to eliminate the malodor naturally.

3. Bad Breath Caused By Smoking

Smoking is a major cause of chronic malodorous breath as a result of the tobacco's smell and also as it makes your gums and teeth vulnerable to disease which leads to bad breath. The best way to eliminate the risk of bad breath because of smoking is to kick the habit as soon as possible.

4. Bad Breath and Dentures

Dentures may also lead to bad breath if they are not cleaned properly. Food particles may get lodged in the dentures and unless cleaned properly, these food particles will aid in the growth of oral bacteria leading to bad breath. This is one of the major reasons that one needs to gargle his mouth properly after every meal.

5. Bad Breath Caused By Dry Mouths

Short – term as well as chronic bad breath can also be caused by dry mouths as the moisture in the mouth helps in keeping it clean.
In a dry mouth, the bacteria can't be moved away. Hence it is advisable to drink the stipulated amount of fluids daily to flush away the oral bacteria. To prevent bad breath, brushing and flossing become mandatory in case of a dry mouth.

The only way to eliminate bad breath is to correctly identify the cause of malodorous breath. Once you've found a cure that successfully deals with bad breath, it will seem like a whole new lease on life.

7 Tips For Curing Bad Breath

One of the most common health problems in society is bad breath. Foul smelling breath might be the effect of variety of reasons. The growth of anaerobic bacteria on the tongue is the most frequent reason for this. The protein present in the food we consume is broken down by these bacteria resulting in the formation of malodorous gases like skatol, hydrogen sulphide etc.

Just about everyone has bad breath when they wake up in the morning. This can be reduced by a significant amount by maintaining good oral hygiene. Some individuals may suffer from bad breath even after they ensure good oral hygiene due to other problems in their mouth or body. Certain diseases also cause bad breath. The precise cause of the bad breath needs to be identified and treated accordingly. Some remedies for bad breath are given below.

1. Good Oral Hygiene

The mouth should be frequently washed to discourage the growth of oral bacteria. Gargling with warm water is vital after every meal. Mouth should be washed even after consuming snacks like sweets or biscuits. Brushing twice a day is necessary. Its is a common adage that brushing in the mornings is for beauty whereas brushing before bedtime is for health.

2. Cleaning the Tongue

Bad breath can also be caused by white or yellow coating on the tongue. This is more prominent I the mornings and has to be removed twice a day with the help of tongue cleaners. Care needs to be taken while using tongue cleaners to prevent the damage to the taste buds.

A tooth pick is basically a small sliver of plastic or wood with a sharp tip. It is used to get rid of particles of food stuck in between the teeth. Its especially useful after consuming meat or fish. It has to be used carefully to avoid damage to the gums.

3. Gargling

Its really useful to gargle the mouth with warm water after every meal. To enhance the effect, salt is added to the water. Various types of mouthwashes are available in the market as well. Using mouthwash to gargle can also reduce the incidence of bad breath.

4. Food Habits

Food rich in proteins is also known to cause bad breath. If food items like meat, fish, milk or eggs are consumed, its vital to clean the mouth properly. Certain food items, like raw onions, have a specific smell which others may find unpleasant. It has been said that an apple a day may keep the doctor away, but a piece of onion a day keeps everyone away. Snack items taken, like nuts, taken between meals may also cause bad breath. Sticking to regular times for meals is vital to avoid bad breath.

5. Drinking Water

A dry mouth forms an ideal environment for the growth of oral bacteria. Saliva is essential to keep the mouth wet and reduce the growth of bacteria. Saliva secretion depends to a large extent on the amount of water consumed and so enough water needs to be drunk to sustain saliva production.

6. Mouth Fresheners

The bad breath can be reduced by using natural or artificial mouth fresheners. Mostly, spicy items are used. Chewing of spices like cumin seed, clove, cinnamon, ginger, garlic etc is also helpful. Citrus fruits also help fight bad breath. Chewing gums and mouth fresheners are available commercially but care needs to be taken in while using them to prevent damage to gums and teeth.

7.Proper Brushing Technique

To avoid bad breadth, good brushing technique is necessary. Brushing vigorously may result in damaged gums. Brushing after every meal and snack could lead to loss of enamel. The bristles of the brush need to be hard but smooth to get rid of particles from between the teeth. The most important aspect of brushing is the direction of brushing. The lower teeth need to brushed

upwards and it's the other way around for the upper teeth. This is valid for both the inner and outer surfaces. For the crowns of the teeth, a forward and backward motion is recommended. This has to be done for both the upper and lower set of teeth.

If none of the above methods work, what can be done?

Try the following -

A. Removal of cause

Bad breath can result from diseases like fevers, diabetes, liver diseases, gastric disorders etc. Removing the primary cause will eliminate the bad breath automatically.

B. Modern Medicine

Bad breath may be caused by an infection and antibiotics, anti-viral and anti-fungal medicine can help cure it. In case it is due to chronic inflammatory conditions or an autoimmune response steroids could be used. Tablets encouraging saliva secretion can also help

C. Dental Cleaning

A visit to the dentist can reduce the amount of plaque and tartar in the mouth. This greatly reduces the intensity of the bad breath.

D. Filling Caries

As caries is one of the major causes of bad breath, it needs to be filled up by a dentist. Initially, silver amalgam was used but now synthetic materials have replaced it. In case the cavity pulp is affected, root canal treatment is needed.

E. Tooth Extraction

In case the caries is deep with major damage to the teeth, extraction of the tooth is the best choice.

F. Tonsillectomy

Patients suffering from chronic tonsillitis can have malodorous breath as a result of the discharges from the crypts of the tonsils. Such people notice a drastic change after tonsillectomy.

G. Psychological Counseling

People suffering from bad breath can become depressed and avoid others. This self inflicted isolation greatly disturbs their normal life. These people need to realize that everybody suffers from bad breath, only their intensity varies. Most people control it by good hygiene. Every has his/her own unique smell which others could find offensive. The need to ensure all personal hygiene is taken care of to reduce the intensity. Psychological support from family and friends is vital.

Certain people visit doctors to cure their bad breath even without a problem. This is considered as somatisation disorder. These people usually suffer from breathlessness, pain, bad breath, abdominal discomfort etc. The presence of any real causes needs to be ruled out with proper diagnosis and psychological support provided for the patient.

H. Homeopathy

Depending on the mental, physical, social and emotional condition of the person, medicine is selected in homeopathy. Depending on the persons constitution, the medicine's strength and dosage is decided. Depending on the coating on the tongue, smell type, cause of bad breath, etc. a medicine is selected. In homeopathy, over 140 medicines are available for bad breath, according to Dr. Robin Murphy. Some of the common drugs used are antim, arnica, sulphur, pulsatilla, nuxvomica, psorinum, etc.

Other homeopathic tinctures like kerosot Q, cinnamon Q, etc. is commonly used for gargling.

Use Science To Answer The Question "How Do I Cure Bad Breath From A High Protein Diet?"

Most people who go on a high protein diet are those who want to build their muscles or those who want to loose weight. Both these categories end up with the problem of bad breath and wonder how to get rid of it. The only way to get rid of this problem is to have a medical consultation and do away with the bad breath once and for all. Both have the problem of building their body mass and loosing weight as soon as possible, so they need professional help to do the right thing with their food habits.

When the food intake is not balanced there are problems
When one is on a fad diet like a high protein one, and the problem of bad breath arises it is obvious that the food intake is not a balanced diet and you would have to correct this to get rid of the bad breath. You may want to burn fat faster but the body's normal parameters also have to be maintained.

There is an accumulation in the blood of ketones once a dieter goes on a high protein diet and this causes bad breath. The body produces ketones when it burns up fat when there are no carbohydrates in the diet. Ketones are expelled from the body in the urine, perspiration and breath. This is the basic cause of bad breath in those who are on a high protein diet.

What is the remedy to give people on a high protein diet with bad breath
The only way and of course the best way is to add on some form of healthy carbohydrates to the daily intake of food. Most people think that high protein is obtained only from sea foods and meats but this is not so. There are many vegetarian foods that give a good protein content to the diet as well as have a certain amount of carbohydrates too. One such very good example is beans which gives a good balance of proteins and carbohydrates so that there the stored fat is not burned up in an incomplete method. Another way to prevent bad breath from a high protein diet is to sweat out the ketones from the pores in the skin, by spending more time in the sun or in saunas instead of from the breath. Drinking a lot of water is another option so that you pass out the ketones in the urine and also dilute those that are in the mouth to prevent bad breath.

Consult a doctor

How To Win Your War Against Bad Breath

To suggest a few basic remedies is alright but in case there is an underlying serious health problem it is better that the person sees a doctor. Undiagnosed diabetes or diabetics who have not got their sugar levels under control could also have bad breath because of ketones that are building up in the blood. This build up of ketones in the blood could prove to be life threatening if not seen to in time.

Laser Zapping Bad Breath

For anyone who has suffered from bad breath, the effects on your self esteem can be devastating. How many times have you been in the close company of others only to wonder if your bad breath was leaving a negative impact? For many people bad breath is a fact of life and, although they have tried my cures, they continue to suffer. Bad breath can be distressing and embarrassing when it occurs every day.

One cause of bad breath, for which there has never before been a cure, is a form of halitosis that emanates from the tonsils. If you're one of these people for whom bad breath is connected to the tonsils you'll be pleased to know that a laser treatment is all that it takes to bring you some relief.

Mild cases of halitosis are usually the result of bacteria in the cavities of the gums or teeth. Bacteria release gases which have a bad odor, such as hydrogen sulphide. To avoid this type of bad breath brush your teeth regularly, use a mouthwash, and make sure that you see your dentist regularly for teeth cleaning.

Certain foods can also cause bad breath in some people in particular strong tasting foods. Garlic is perhaps the number one culprit of bad breath and can leave a lingering smell that can last for several hours. Other foods that can cause bad breath include strong spices, cabbage, and alcohol.

Your tonsils can also be a cause of your bad breath. This is because your tonsils have grooves and pits that are perfect places for anaerobic bacteria to thrive in. The good news is that there is now a laser procedure available that can help to seal these grooves in your tonsils so that bacteria can no longer enter. The entire procedure will take about fifteen minutes from beginning to end.

The laser is used to vaporize the tonsil tissue that is infected so that scar tissue is created. Bacteria will be unable to penetrate this scar tissue and therefore have no place to breed. Most patients will be cured of their bad breath after just one laser treatment while other patients will need to have two or three treatments.

How To Win Your War Against Bad Breath

Before you try laser treatment for your bad breath you'll want to try more conventional methods of treatment first. This includes using mouthwash, brushing your teeth more often, or scraping the tongue. If nothing else seems to work, contact your doctor or dentist to find out more information about laser treatment for bad breath.

Fighting Bad Breath From A Low Carb Diet

You may find that you lose a lot of weight when you're on a low carb diet but one of the side effects of this weight loss is bad breath. Many dentists are finding that they get a lot of complaints from their patients about bad breath. Patients think that it might be tooth decay that is causing them to have foul breath but, after a dental exam, dentists find that tooth decay isn't an issue. This bad breath is actually called "ketone breath" and has a sweet sick smell to it. Ketone breath is the result of chemicals built in the body due to a low carb diet.

Low carb diets work when your body burns up stored fat as a fuel rather than using carbohydrates. When your body fat is burned up as fuel smelly ketones, or chemicals, are built up in the body. These ketone chemicals are then released in your urine and in your breath. Hence, bad breath is one of the biggest side effects of a low carb diet.

Many times bad breath will occur during the breakdown of certain food particles which have sulphur components. Bacteria found on the tongue and gums are another culprit. Foods that are high in protein will produce large amounts of sulphur compounds particularly at night when there is less saliva to wash away these components.

There a few **things that you can do to battle "ketone breath"** if you're on a low carb diet:

- Make sure that you drink plenty of water so that you wash away the bacteria and germs in your mouth.
- Chew on fresh pieces of parsley
- Chew sugarless gum.
- Take the time to brush your teeth and tongue every time you eat.
- Take the time to floss after every meal.
- Try bleaching your teeth. Bleaching can help against bad breath because it acts as an oxygenating agent that kills germs and bacteria.

Bad breath can have a negative impact on almost anything that you do in your day from talking to co-workers to kissing your partner. When you're trying to lose weight, the last thing that you want to do is focus on your breath when you want to start feeling better about yourself. The

How To Win Your War Against Bad Breath

above tips can help you keep a lid on bad breath so that you can put your energies into your weight loss program.

If you find that your bad breath continues after you've finished your low carb diet, make sure that you see a doctor. Bad breath can be a sign of serious medical conditions such as diabetes.

How To Get Rid Of Bad Breath For Good

People who suffer from bad breath know the misery of it, and they are willing to do anything to learn how to get rid of bad breath. The good news is that you can easily learn how to get rid of bad breath, given that the condition is not due to a medical condition. You simply need to observe the food that you eat and maintain hygienic oral conditions on a regular basis.

What Causes Bad Breath?

Commonly, food particles get stuck in between your teeth after you have eaten and give rise to bad breath. People who take protein-rich diets are the ones who usually face this problem, and they have to literally struggle to learn how to get rid of bad breath. On the contrary, people who eat plenty of fresh fruits and vegetables hardly need to bother about learning how to get rid of bad breath. Fresh fruits and vegetables give rise to a fresh and clean breath. No wonder we hardly see vegetarians struggling to learn how to get rid of bad breath.

Five Simple Ways to Get Rid of Bad Breath

An average person can easily learn how to get rid of bad breath, provided he or she is not suffering from a gastric disorder or some other medical condition. The chief agents that cause bad breath are the bacteria that feed on the food sticking to your teeth. Follow these five simple points that teach you how to get rid of bad breath.

First and foremost, invest in a good toothbrush and some floss. This is the best way you can learn how to get rid of bad breath. It is very important that you pay special attention to oral hygiene.

Second, learn to brush your tongue in addition to brushing your teeth if you want to get rid of bad breath permanently. The bacteria that love feasting on the food stuck to your teeth also enjoy burrowing into your tongue. Drive them away by regularly brushing your tongue. Now, you are on the way to learning how to get rid of bad breath.

Third, fix a convenient schedule for oral hygiene. This practice will get rid of all the bacteria responsible for your bad breath. Brush your teeth after every meal and floss regularly. Using a

How To Win Your War Against Bad Breath

disinfectant mouthwash will flush out from your mouth all the bacterial culprits that are responsible for your bad breath.

Fourth, quit smoking for good because it is the number one cause of bad breath. If you are smoker, the cigarette smoke will lend a bad smell not only your mouth, but also your clothes and hair. Dental equipment such as toothpaste, floss, and mouthwash might control bad breath in case of smokers; however, they can do nothing about the bad smell arising from a smoker's body. If you want to really get rid of bad breath, seriously consider quitting smoking for good.

Fifth, stop drinking alcoholic beverages because they can give you a bad breath. If you are a heavy drinker, your breath will smell of alcohol. Even if you try all methods available under the sun, including the use of mouth fresheners, you will not be successful in getting rid of the smell.

Bad Breath In Children

If your child has bad breath you'll want to get to the bottom of the problem so that you can rule out health problems. Most bad breath in children is the result of tooth decay. As soon as your child's teeth appear they are susceptible to decay. This means that you have to practice good dental hygiene habits from a very young age, as early as the first birthday. Get a soft brush and brush your child's teeth after nursing or after a bottle. When you start introducing foods to you child's diet make sure that you take the time to brush lightly so that food particles are removed from the mouth. Never put your child to bed with a bottle since this is the number one leading cause of tooth decay.

If teeth aren't the problem behind bad breath in your child other health problems might be. Other health issues can include throat problems, sinus infections, or an obstruction from the adenoids or tonsils. After children have a cold they are often susceptible to respiratory conditions which can produce bad breath.

Certain food groups can also cause bad breath in children. Try eliminating foods in groups for about two to four weeks to see if your child's breath improves. Some of the food groups to eliminate include dairy, wheat and other glutens, citrus, shellfish, and eggs.

Bad Breath In Dogs

Bad breath isn't just something that people experience. Having a pet with bad breath can make your life very uncomfortable. Some of the common reasons for bad breath in dogs are caused by gum and tooth problems. However, bad breath in dogs can also be an indication of other health problems. The important thing to do is determine why your dog has breath that is less than pleasant.

Dogs will often develop a build up of tartar around their teeth. After eating, particles of food will remain in your dog's mouth. These particles will start to decompose and it's this decomposition that will create a great environment for bacteria to thrive. The bacteria will then multiply to form plaque. Plaque is a combination of decomposed foods, minerals, and bacteria. And it's the plaque that will affect your dog's dental hygiene and cause him to have bad breath. Plaque is the leading cause of tooth loss for dogs since it will stick to the bottom of the teeth, causing the gums to recede and become inflamed.

When your dog is affected by plaque you'll find that he eats less. During the early stages of plaque disease there will be a yellow or brown coating on the sides of the teeth particularly around the large molar teeth. Smaller breeds of dogs seem to have more problems with plaque than larger breed dogs. Good dental hygiene is essential for dogs so that plaque doesn't have a chance to develop. Make sure that your give your dog an annual dental examine. You'll be saving his teeth as well as avoiding bad breath.

There are other causes of bad breath in dogs besides plaque. When your dog is shedding his baby teeth you may find that he drools and has bad breath. This bad breath problem will disappear when all of the baby teeth have been replaced by adult teeth. During this stage of your dog's life you can brush his mouth with a solution of diluted baking soda and water. This will give your dog some relief from teething pain as well as freshen his breath.

Older dogs may have medical conditions that can affect their breath. This includes liver and kidney problems. A dog with these medical problems will be very thin and have a small appetite. Your vet will be able to determine if your dog's bad breath is a symptom of organ failure. Your dog's teeth will need to be cleaned and a course of antibiotics administered to be sure that infection doesn't set in.

How To Win Your War Against Bad Breathing

This Product Is Brought To You By

DAVID A OSEI

www.ingramcontent.com/pod-product-compliance
Lightning Source LLC
Chambersburg PA
CBHW051228250726
48655CB00006B/2663